THE HAIR CARE HANDBOOK

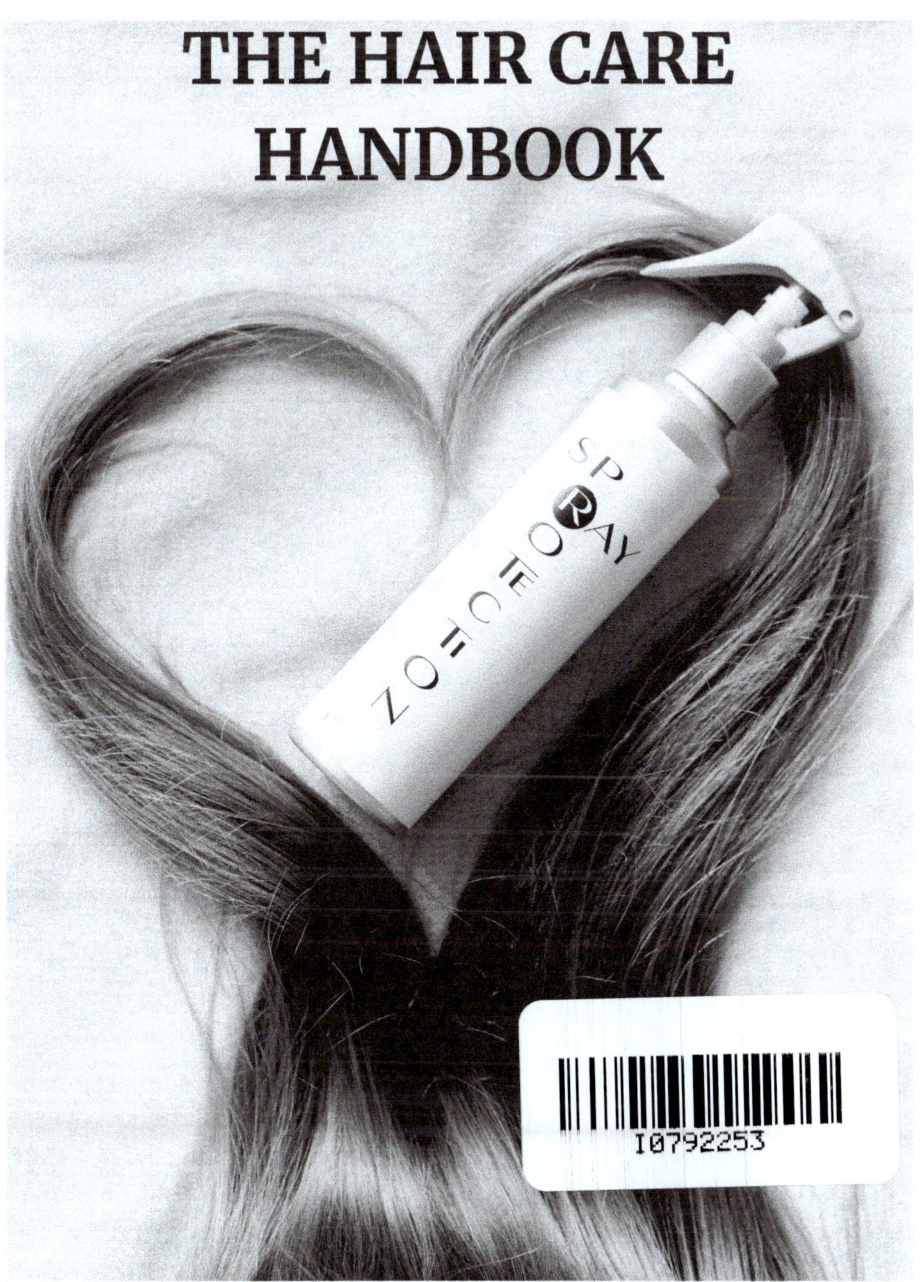

SECRETS TO GORGEOUS, STRONG, AND LUSCIOUS LOCKS

CONTENTS OF THE BOOK:

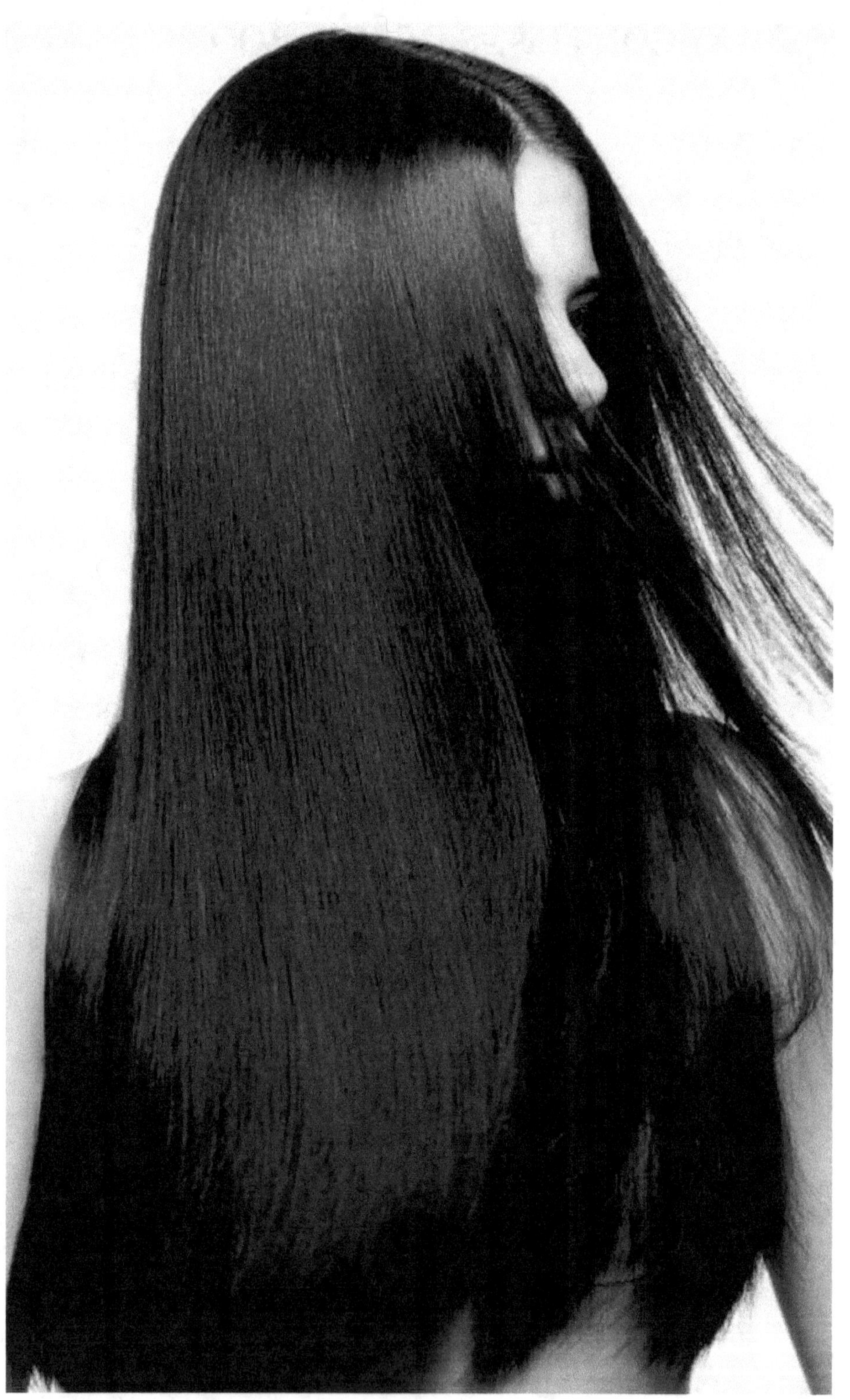

INTRODUCTION

Every woman deserves to feel confident, radiant, and powerful—and nothing completes that feeling like a crown of gorgeous hair. Whether your hair is sleek and straight, soft and wavy, or full of curls and coils, it tells a story about who you are. But achieving hair that feels healthy, strong, and beautiful doesn't have to be a mystery.

Welcome to The Hair Care Handbook, your ultimate companion on the journey to stunning locks. This book is packed with the knowledge, tools, and tips you need to understand your hair's unique needs and care for it like never before. From the science of hair growth to tailored routines, natural remedies, and solutions for common challenges, every chapter is designed to empower you to create a hair care regimen that works for your life and your goals.

In these pages, you'll discover:

- How to understand your hair's structure and type, and why this is key to its health.
- The secrets behind hair growth and how to encourage it naturally.
- Remedies for damage, frizz, and thinning, so you can overcome challenges with confidence.
- DIY treatments and natural recipes that you

can make at home for a touch of luxury and effectiveness.

- Tips for choosing the right products and creating a routine that's simple yet powerful.

Whether you're just beginning your hair care journey or looking to refine your current routine, this book will help you make informed choices that bring out the very best in your hair. Along the way, you'll learn that taking care of your hair isn't just about appearance—it's a form of self-love and care that brings balance and joy to your life.

Your hair is unique, and so is your journey. Let's embrace it together, step by step, as we uncover the secrets to gorgeous, strong, and luscious locks. Your best hair days are ahead—and they start right here.

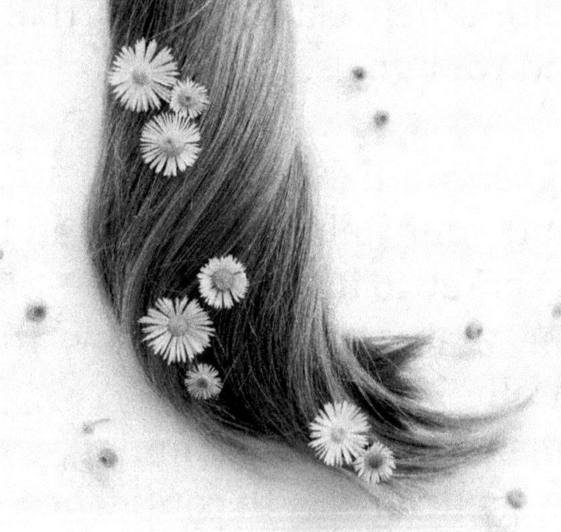

CHAPTER 1: THE SECRETS TO UNDERSTANDING AND NURTURING YOUR HAIR

Every woman dreams of having hair that feels like a crown—strong, shiny, and full of life. But the first step to unlocking the secrets to beautiful, healthy, thick hair lies in understanding it. Hair isn't just about beauty; it's an extension of who you are, and like anything valuable, it needs proper care and love. Let's dive into the essentials of hair structure, care, and how to tailor your routine to suit your unique locks.

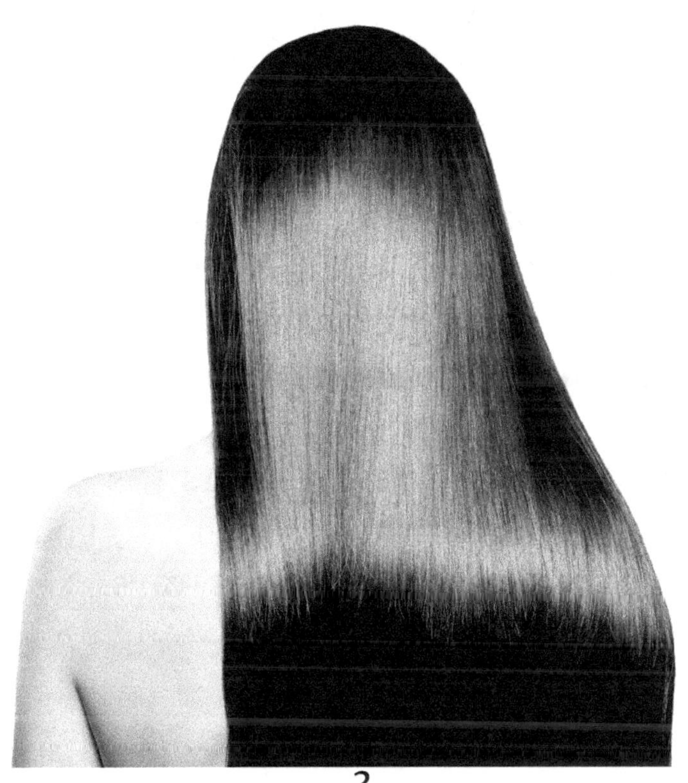

The Structure of Hair: Your Hair's Hidden World

At a glance, hair might seem simple, but each strand is a marvel of nature. Hair has three main layers:

- The Cuticle: This is the outermost layer and acts as a shield for the inner layers. Think of it as the armor that protects your hair. When healthy, the cuticle lies flat, reflecting light and giving your hair that enviable shine.

- The Cortex: Beneath the cuticle lies the cortex, the powerhouse of your hair. It's responsible for strength, color, and elasticity. Whether your hair bounces back after being pulled or maintains its color, it's thanks to the cortex.

- The Medulla: The innermost core of the hair, the medulla, is mostly found in thicker hair and doesn't significantly impact hair's strength or appearance.

- Understanding these layers is essential because every product or habit you adopt interacts with them in unique ways.

Basic Rules for Beautiful Hair Care

Regardless of your hair type, there are golden rules every woman should follow to keep her tresses healthy and happy:

Cleanse with Care: Overwashing can strip hair of natural oils, leaving it dry and brittle. Aim for 2-3 washes a week, using a sulfate-free shampoo to gently cleanse without damaging the cuticle.

Condition for Protection: Conditioner isn't just an optional step; it's a must. It smooths the cuticle and locks in moisture. Focus on the ends, where your hair tends to be the driest.

Avoid Heat Overload: Frequent heat styling can weaken the cortex, causing split ends and breakage. When possible, let your hair air dry or use a heat protectant when styling.

Nourish from Within: Healthy hair starts with a balanced diet rich in vitamins like Biotin, Vitamin E, and Omega-3 fatty acids. Don't underestimate the power of hydration—drink plenty of water for both your skin and scalp.

Regular Trims Are Key: A trim every 6-8 weeks prevents split ends from traveling up the shaft, preserving your hair's health and thickness.

Caring for Different Hair Types

Each type of hair—straight, wavy, curly, or coily—has unique needs. Tailoring your routine to your specific hair type ensures it thrives:

Straight Hair: Straight hair tends to get oily faster because natural oils travel down the shaft more easily. Use a lightweight shampoo and avoid heavy products that can weigh it down.

Wavy Hair: Wavy hair benefits from hydration without overloading. Use leave-in conditioners or lightweight creams to enhance waves while preventing frizz.

Curly Hair: Curly hair craves moisture due to its structure, which makes it harder for oils to travel down the strands. Opt for deep conditioning treatments weekly and avoid harsh brushing.

Coily Hair: Coily hair is the most fragile of all types, requiring extra TLC. Incorporate nourishing oils like argan or jojoba into your routine and use protective styles to minimize breakage.

Your Scalp: The Root of Healthy Hair

Beautiful hair begins at the roots—literally. A healthy scalp creates the foundation for strong, thick hair. Avoid using products that can clog your scalp, like heavy pomades, and incorporate a gentle exfoliating scrub once a month to remove buildup. Scalp massages with nourishing oils improve blood circulation and encourage hair growth.

The Journey to Your Dream Hair

Hair care is a journey, not a sprint. Be patient with your routine, and remember that consistency is more important than perfection. The key to beautiful hair is understanding its needs and nurturing it with love.

In the next chapter, we'll explore the science of hair growth and how to create a personalized hair care plan to suit your lifestyle and goals. Until then, treat every strand like a treasure—it deserves it!

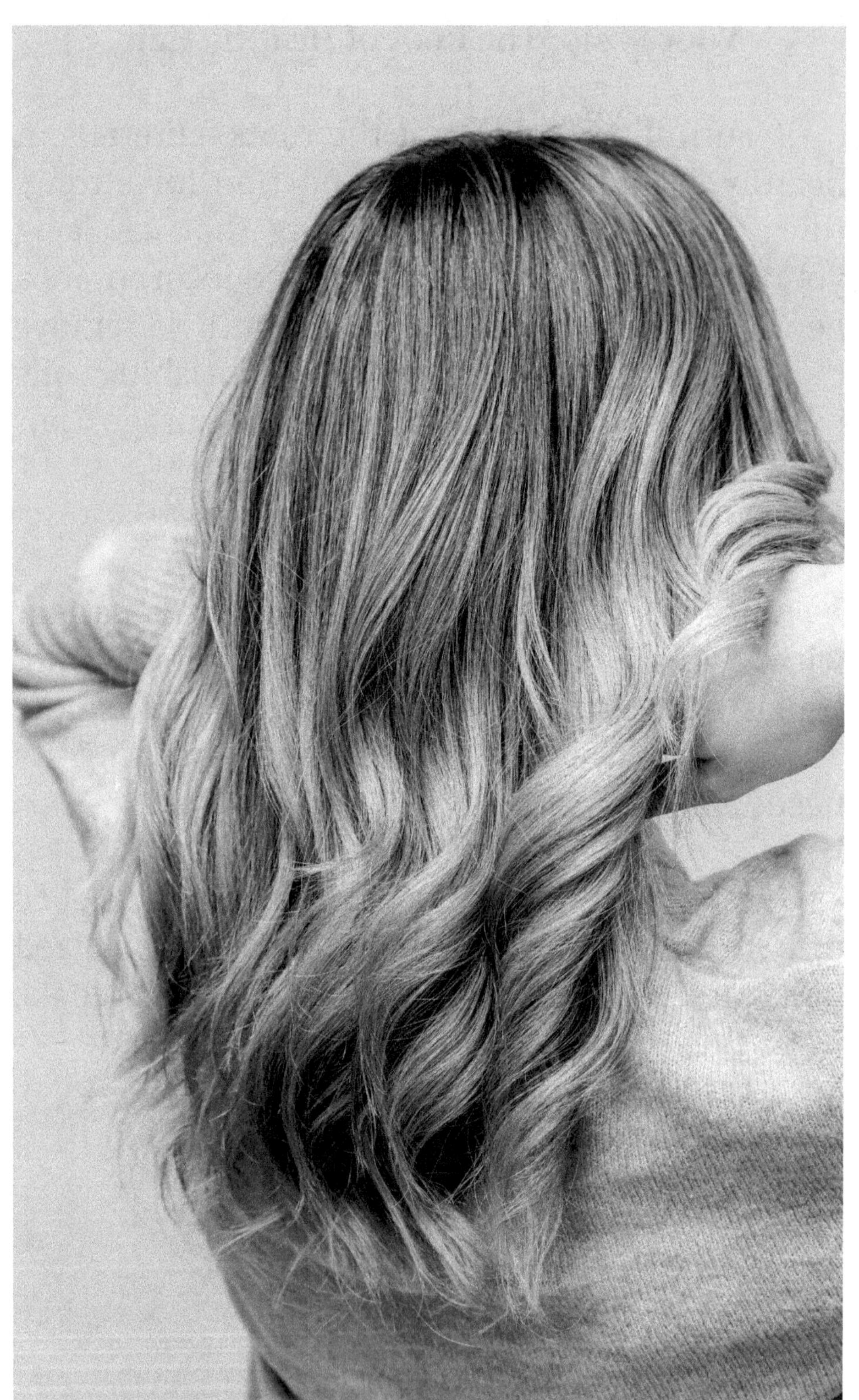

CHAPTER 2: GROWING GLORY—YOUR PERSONALIZED PATH TO HEALTHY, LUSH HAIR

Your hair grows every day—it's a silent, fascinating process happening right on your head! But how can you support your hair's natural growth and make sure every strand is strong and vibrant? In this chapter, we'll unravel the mysteries of hair growth and help you create a hair care plan tailored to your lifestyle and goals. Plus, we'll explore vitamins, products, and techniques that can boost growth and improve your hair's overall condition.

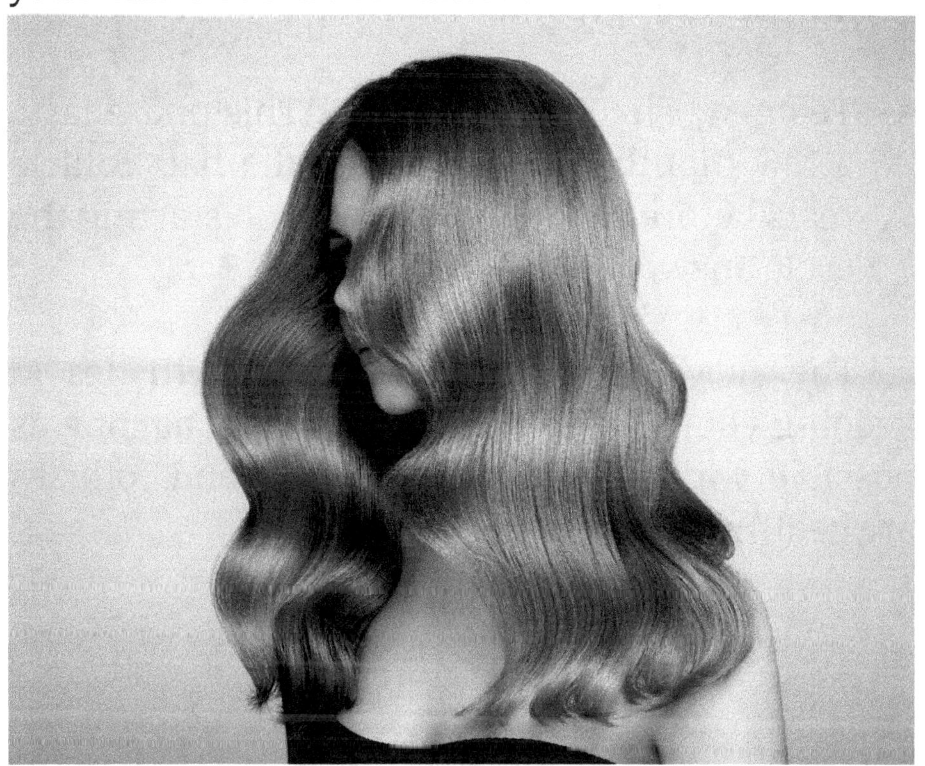

The Science of Hair Growth

Hair growth is a cycle—a continuous dance between phases that keep your locks evolving. There are three main stages:

- Anagen (The Growth Phase): This is when your hair actively grows, and it can last anywhere from 2 to 7 years depending on your genetics. The longer this phase, the longer your hair can grow!

- Catagen (The Transition Phase): A short period of about 2-3 weeks where growth slows and the hair prepares to shed.

- Telogen (The Resting Phase): This phase lasts a few months, during which the hair follicle rests before shedding the hair and starting the cycle anew.

The key to promoting hair growth lies in keeping your hair in the anagen phase as long as possible while ensuring your scalp and follicles are healthy.

Creating Your Personalized Hair Care Plan

Every woman's hair journey is unique, and your hair care routine should reflect your lifestyle, time, and goals. Here's a step-by-step guide to designing your ideal plan:

Step 1: Define Your Goals

Do you want longer hair, more volume, less breakage, or just overall health? Be clear about what you're working toward so you can choose the right methods and products.

Step 2: Assess Your Lifestyle

Busy Schedule: Choose low-maintenance routines, like overnight treatments or weekly deep conditioning.

Active Lifestyle: Use products that protect your hair from sweat and frequent washing, like clarifying shampoos and lightweight conditioners.

Frequent Heat Styling: Incorporate a high-quality heat protectant and repair products to counteract damage.

Step 3: Customize Your Routine

Daily Care: Focus on gentle detangling, hydration, and scalp care.

Weekly Care: Include deep conditioning, scalp

exfoliation, or a hair mask tailored to your hair type.

Monthly Care: Trim split ends and evaluate your routine to see what's working.

Vitamins for Hair Growth

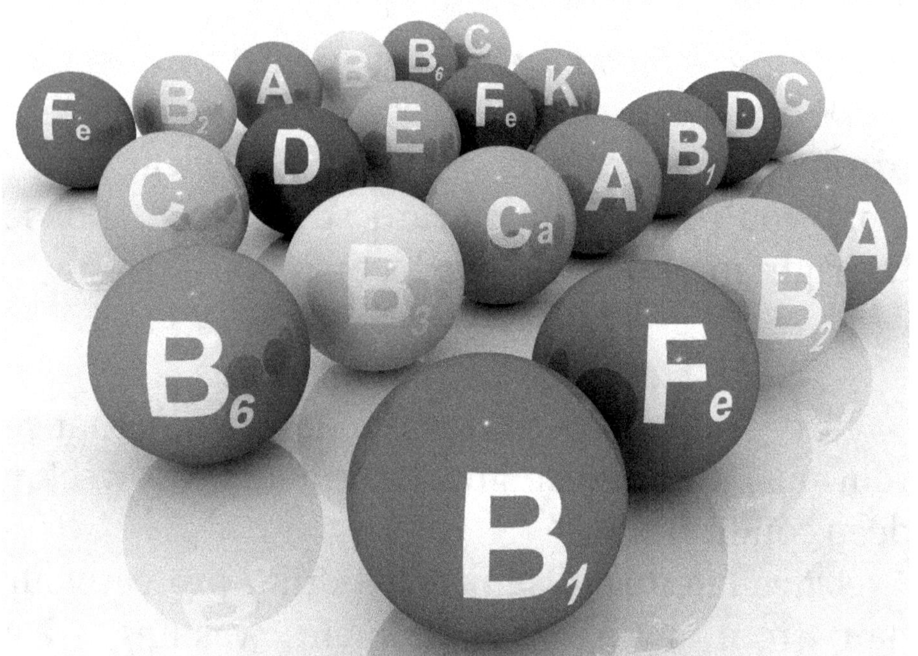

Healthy hair starts from within! Your body needs the right nutrients to support growth, and these powerhouse vitamins and minerals can help:

Biotin (Vitamin B7):   Known as the "hair vitamin," biotin strengthens the structure of your hair, making it less prone to breakage. It's found in foods like eggs, nuts, and avocados.

Vitamin D: Essential for stimulating hair follicles, Vitamin D deficiency can slow hair growth. Get it through sunlight, fortified foods, or supplements.

Vitamin E: This antioxidant improves scalp circulation and supports hair growth. Nuts, seeds, and spinach are great sources.

Iron: A lack of iron can lead to hair thinning. Incorporate lean meats, spinach, and lentils into your diet.

Omega-3 Fatty Acids: Found in fish like salmon and walnuts, these healthy fats keep your scalp moisturized and reduce inflammation that could stunt growth.

Tip: Supplements can be helpful, but always check with a healthcare provider before starting any new regimen to ensure they suit your needs.

You can find more about vitamins in my book: "The Power of Vitamins: Understanding Vitamins and Their Role in Your Life".

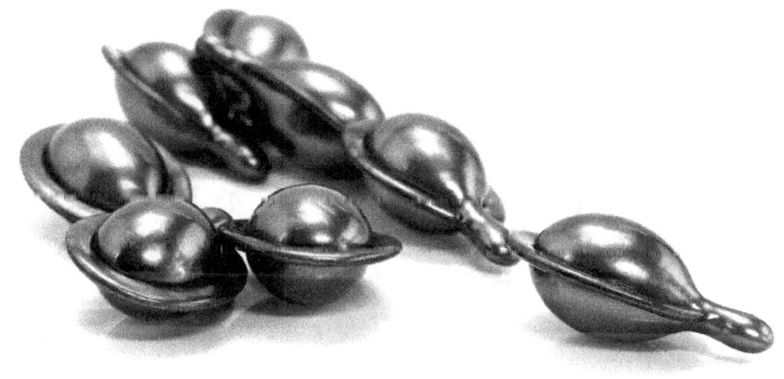

Products That Support Hair Growth

The market is filled with products claiming to grow your hair faster, but which ones actually work? Here's what to look for:

Scalp Serums: Look for ingredients like caffeine, niacinamide, or peppermint oil, which boost circulation to the scalp and stimulate follicles.

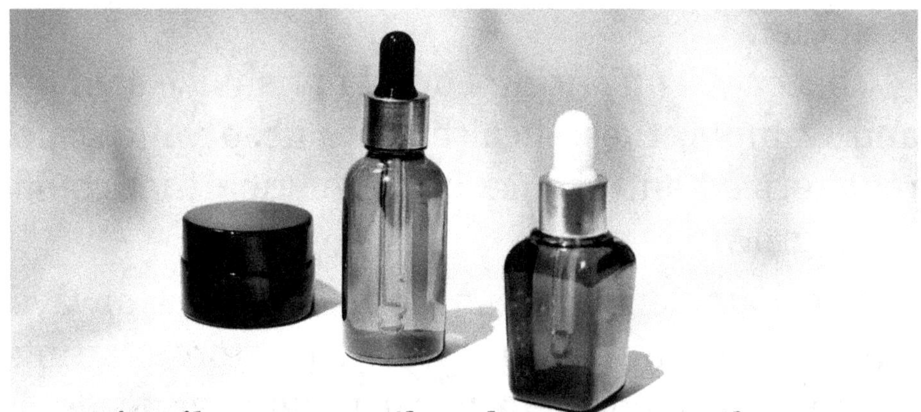

Hair Oils: Castor oil and rosemary oil are stars for promoting growth. Apply them as a scalp treatment before washing your hair.

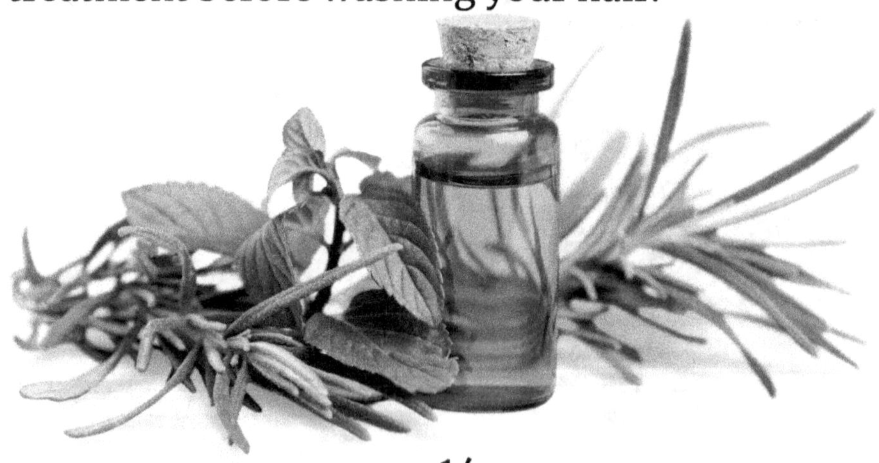

Shampoos and Conditioners: Opt for sulfate-free formulas that include keratin, biotin, or collagen to strengthen and nourish your strands.

Leave-in Treatments: Lightweight sprays or creams with heat protection and vitamins can protect hair throughout the day.

Lifestyle Habits for Better Growth

Hair health isn't just about what you put on your hair—it's also about your daily habits:

Sleep on Satin: Cotton pillowcases can cause friction and breakage. Switch to satin or silk to keep your hair smooth.

Reduce Stress: Stress can lead to hair shedding. Incorporate relaxation techniques like yoga, meditation, or simply taking time for self-care.

Stay Hydrated: Water hydrates every cell in your body, including your hair follicles. Make it a habit to drink water throughout the day.

Patience: The Final Ingredient

Hair growth is a slow process—on average, hair grows about half an inch per month. While it's easy to feel impatient, remember that consistency is more important than speed. Every small effort, from eating better to massaging your scalp, adds up over time.

In the next chapter, we'll tackle the common challenges of hair care—dealing with damage, frizz, and thinning—and how to restore your hair to its full potential. For now, keep nurturing your hair with love and care, and watch as it grows into the beautiful, thick crown you've always dreamed of!

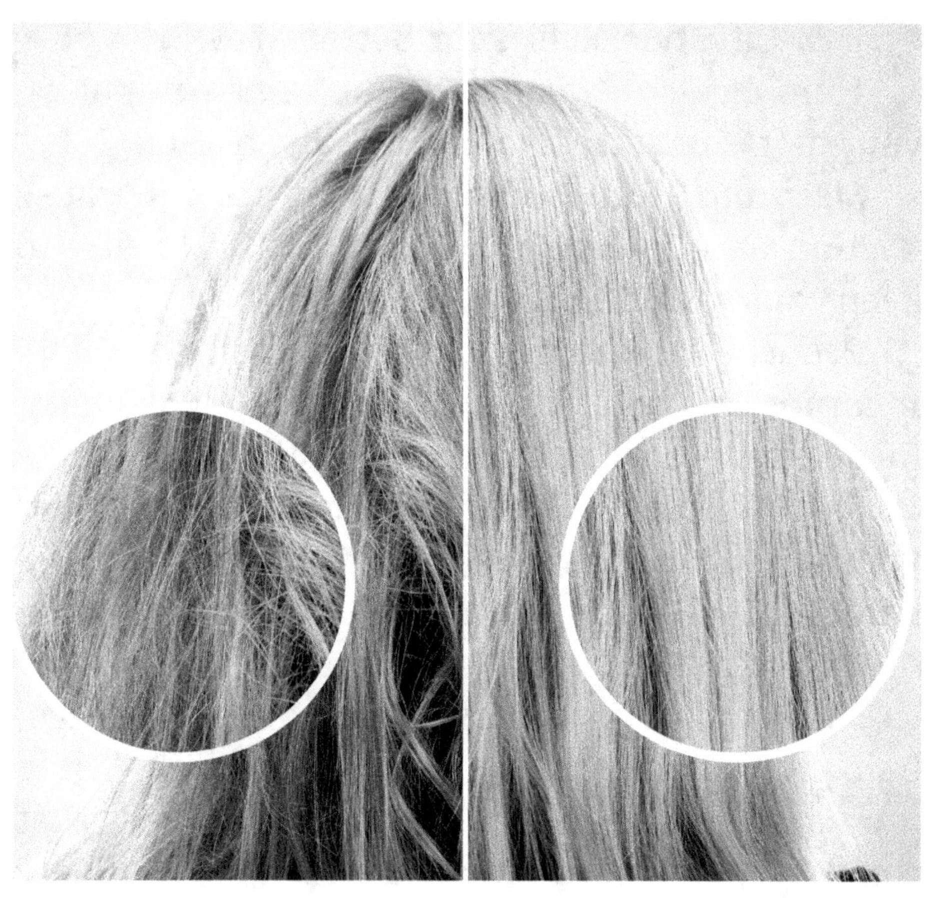

CHAPTER 3: OVERCOMING HAIR CARE CHALLENGES—YOUR PATH TO HEALTHY, RESILIENT HAIR

No matter how much care we give, our hair can face challenges that seem to stand in the way of achieving our dream locks. Damage, frizz, and thinning are among the most common issues women encounter, but the good news is they're not permanent. Hair has an incredible ability to bounce back when given the right care and attention. In this chapter, we'll identify the causes of these problems and explore practical solutions to help your hair reach its full, healthy potential.

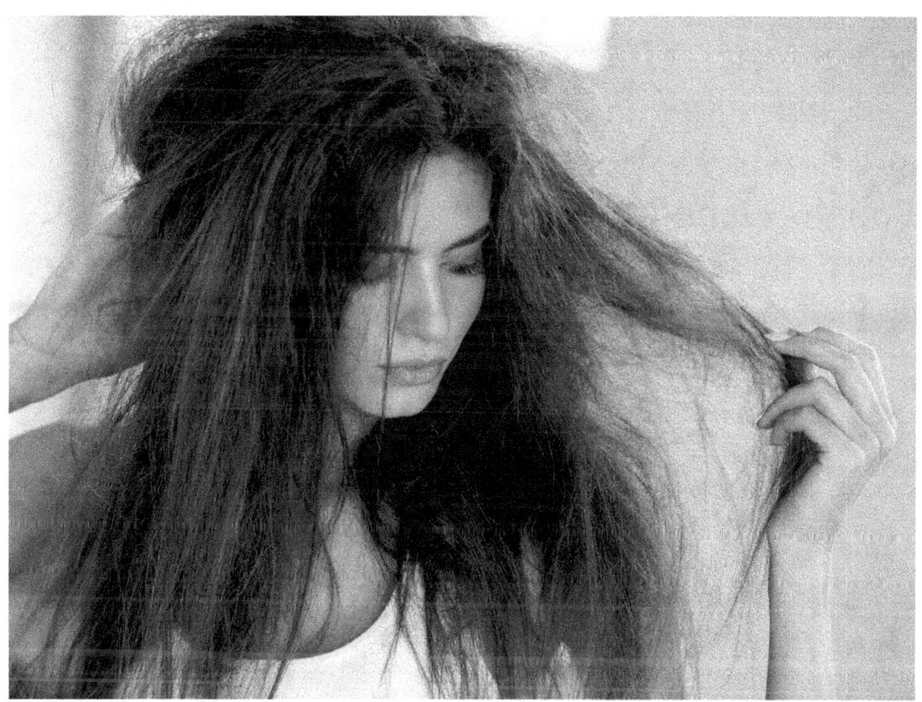

Understanding Hair Damage
What does damaged hair look like?

Split ends, dullness, rough texture, and breakage are all signs of damage. This happens when the cuticle (the protective outer layer of your hair) is worn down, leaving the cortex vulnerable.

What causes damage?

Heat Styling: Frequent use of flat irons, curling wands, and blow dryers can weaken hair over time.

Chemical Treatments: Coloring, bleaching, and perms break down the structure of your hair to achieve their effects.

Environmental Stress: Sun exposure, pollution, and harsh weather can strip hair of its moisture.
Rough Handling: Tugging, over-brushing, or using the wrong tools can contribute to breakage.

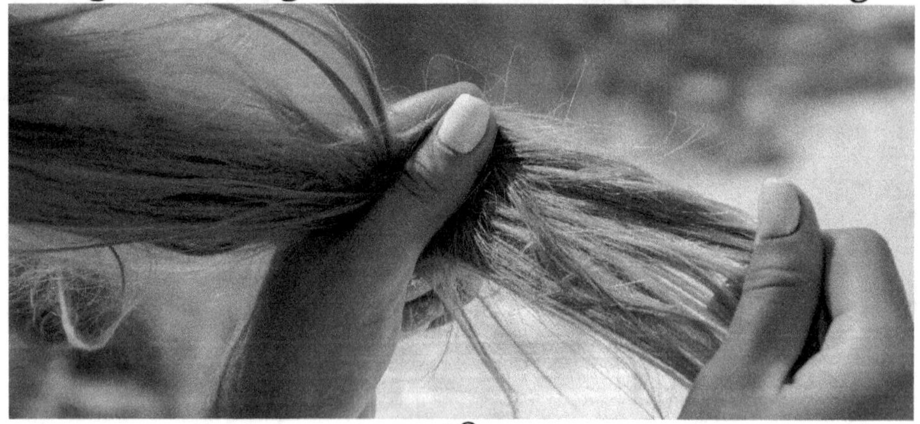

How can you restore damaged hair?

Hydrate Deeply: Use a deep conditioning mask weekly to restore moisture and repair the cuticle. Look for masks with keratin, argan oil, or shea butter.

Trim the Damage: Regular trims are essential to get rid of split ends, preventing them from traveling up the hair shaft.

Use Heat Sparingly: Give your hair a break from heat tools and always apply a heat protectant when styling.

Reinforce with Protein: If your hair feels limp or breaks easily, it may need protein. Use treatments labeled as "protein reconstructors," but don't overdo it—too much protein can make hair stiff.

Conquering Frizz

Why does frizz happen?

Frizz is your hair's way of crying out for moisture. It occurs when the cuticle lifts, allowing humidity to penetrate and swell the strands.

What causes frizz?

Dryness: When hair lacks moisture, it tries to pull it from the air, causing frizz.

Humidity: Excess moisture in the air disrupts the balance of your hair.

Improper Drying: Rubbing your hair with a towel or air-drying in humid environments can make frizz worse.

How can you tame frizz?

Hydration is Key: Use a hydrating shampoo and conditioner. Ingredients like glycerin and hyaluronic acid draw moisture into the hair.

Seal the Cuticle: Finish your routine with a lightweight serum or leave-in conditioner to smooth the cuticle and lock out humidity.

Dry Gently: Instead of rubbing your hair with a towel, pat it dry with a microfiber towel or an old T-shirt.

Style Smart: Opt for hairstyles that work with your hair's natural texture instead of fighting against it. Braids, buns, or twists can keep frizz at bay.

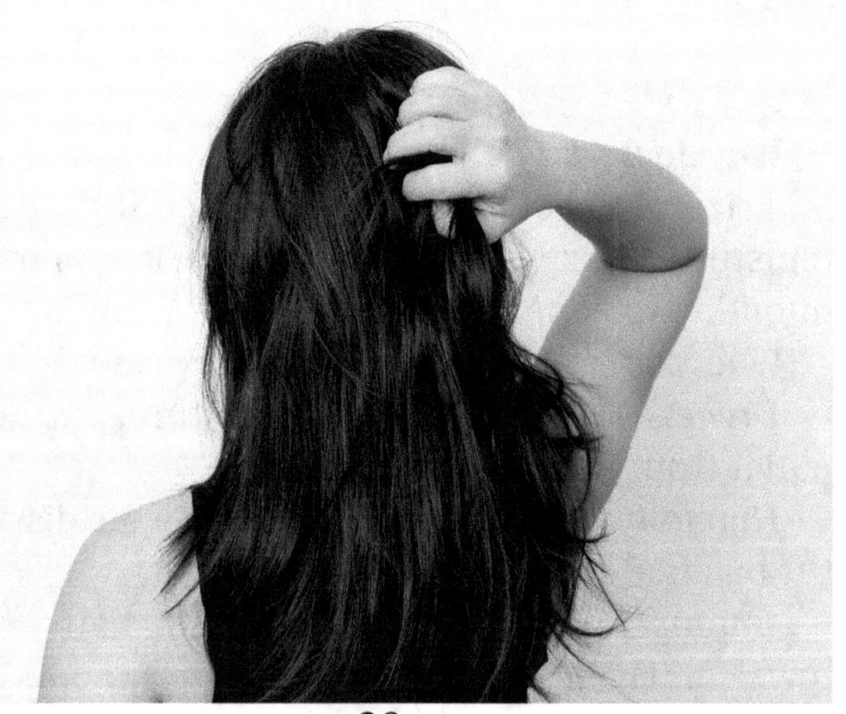

Addressing Thinning Hair

What causes thinning?

Thinning hair can be caused by several factors, including:

Stress: Chronic stress disrupts the hair growth cycle, causing more strands to enter the shedding phase.

Hormonal Changes: Pregnancy, menopause, or conditions like polycystic ovary syndrome (PCOS) can affect hair growth.

Nutritional Deficiencies: Lack of key nutrients like iron, biotin, and zinc can weaken hair follicles.

Aging: Over time, hair naturally becomes finer and grows more slowly.

How can you restore volume?

Stimulate the Scalp: Regular scalp massages with oils like rosemary or peppermint improve blood circulation and encourage hair growth.

Check Your Diet: Ensure you're eating a balanced diet rich in protein, vitamins, and healthy fats. Foods like salmon, eggs, and leafy greens are hair-boosting superstars.

Use Targeted Treatments: Hair growth serums with ingredients like minoxidil or peptides can help strengthen thinning hair.

Handle Hair Gently: Avoid tight hairstyles that

pull on the scalp and use a wide-tooth comb to detangle without breakage.

Tips to Prevent Hair Problems Before They Start

Protect Your Hair at Night: Sleeping on a silk or satin pillowcase reduces friction and helps hair retain moisture.

Be Sun-Savvy: Protect your hair from UV damage by wearing a hat or using hair products with built-in SPF.

Limit Washing: Washing hair too often strips it of natural oils. Aim for every 2-3 days unless you have an oily scalp.

Choose the Right Products: Avoid sulfates, parabens, and alcohol in hair care products, as they can be drying.

Embrace the Process

Hair challenges can be frustrating, but every issue is an opportunity to learn more about your hair and how to care for it better. By understanding the root cause of damage, frizz, or thinning, you're already on the path to healthier, stronger, and more beautiful locks.

In the next chapter, we'll explore how to elevate your hair care routine with DIY treatments and natural remedies you can whip up in your own kitchen. Remember, your hair is unique—just like you—and with a little care and patience, it can thrive like never before.

CHAPTER 4: THE MAGIC OF DIY HAIR CARE—25 NATURAL RECIPES FOR GORGEOUS HAIR

There's something special about using simple, natural ingredients to care for your hair. These remedies, straight from your kitchen, are often more effective than expensive store-bought products—and they're free of harsh chemicals. In this chapter, we'll explore how to use homemade treatments to nourish your hair, improve its growth, and leave it looking and feeling its best. Plus, you'll find 25 easy-to-make recipes for hair masks tailored to different needs.

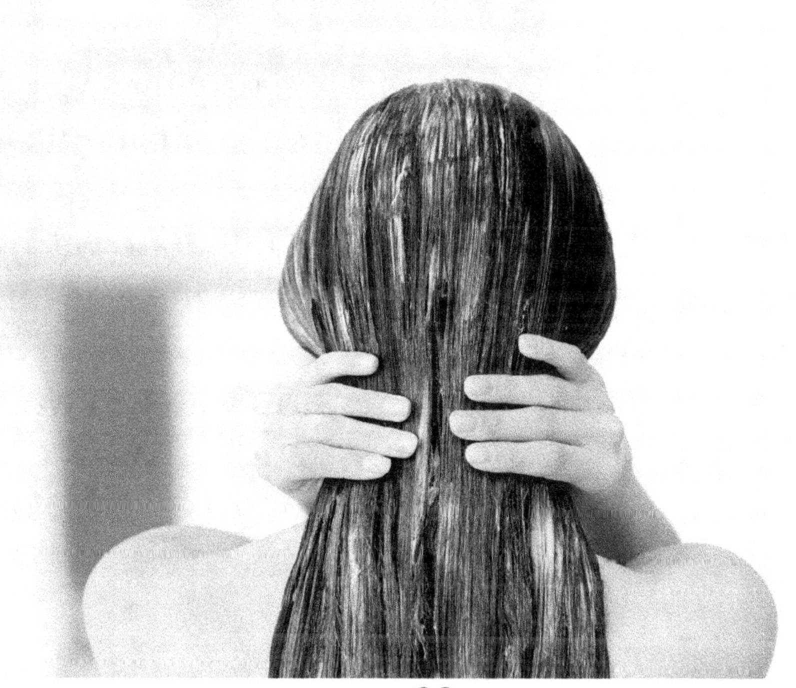

Why Choose DIY Hair Care?

Homemade treatments are a way to reconnect with nature and give your hair the love it deserves. They offer:

Customization: You can create recipes tailored to your hair type and specific concerns.

Purity: No hidden chemicals or artificial fragrances—just pure, natural goodness.

Affordability: Many remedies use common pantry items, making them cost-effective.

How to Use Homemade Hair Treatments

Start with Clean Hair: Apply masks to freshly washed, towel-dried hair to allow nutrients to penetrate deeply.

Don't Overdo It: Once a week is usually enough for most treatments, though some can be used more often.

Cover for Best Results: Wrap your hair with a shower cap or warm towel to lock in heat and enhance absorption.

Rinse Thoroughly: Use lukewarm water to wash out the mask, followed by a gentle shampoo if needed.

25 RECIPES FOR HEALTHY, BEAUTIFUL HAIR

FOR DEEP MOISTURE AND REPAIR

- Avocado and Olive Oil Mask: Mash ½ an avocado with 2 tbsp olive oil. Apply for 20 minutes to restore shine and softness.
- Banana and Honey Mask: Blend 1 ripe banana with 1 tbsp honey. This ultra-moisturizing mask smooths frizz and repairs dryness.
- Yogurt and Aloe Vera Mask: Combine ½ cup plain yogurt with 3 tbsp aloe vera gel for hydration and scalp soothing.
- Coconut Milk and Vitamin E Mask: Mix ½ cup coconut milk with the contents of a Vitamin E capsule to nourish dry, damaged hair.
- Shea Butter and Argan Oil Mask: Melt 2 tbsp shea butter and mix with 1 tbsp argan oil for a luxurious treatment.

FOR HAIR GROWTH AND STRENGTH

- Castor Oil and Rosemary Mask: Combine 2 tbsp castor oil with 5 drops of rosemary essential oil. Massage into the scalp to stimulate growth.
- Egg and Lemon Mask: Beat 1 egg with the juice of half a lemon to strengthen hair and reduce shedding.

- Onion Juice and Coconut Oil Mask: Mix 3 tbsp onion juice with 1 tbsp coconut oil to boost circulation and growth.
- Green Tea Rinse: Brew a strong cup of green tea and use it as a rinse after shampooing to stimulate follicles.
- Rice Water Rinse: Soak rice in water for 30 minutes, strain, and use the water as a growth-boosting rinse.

FOR SCALP HEALTH

- Apple Cider Vinegar Rinse: Dilute 2 tbsp apple cider vinegar in 1 cup of water to balance scalp pH and remove buildup.
- Fenugreek and Yogurt Mask: Soak 2 tbsp fenugreek seeds overnight, blend into a paste, and mix with yogurt for a dandruff-fighting scalp treatment.
- Neem and Coconut Oil Mask: Blend fresh neem leaves with 2 tbsp coconut oil for an antimicrobial treatment.
- Honey and Cinnamon Mask: Mix 2 tbsp honey with 1 tsp cinnamon powder to improve blood flow and scalp health.
- Aloe Vera and Peppermint Oil Mask: Blend 3 tbsp aloe vera gel with 3 drops of peppermint oil to cool and invigorate the scalp.

- Honey and Coconut Oil Mask: Combine 2 tbsp honey with 2 tbsp coconut oil for a glossy finish.
- Apple and Cucumber Mask: Blend half an apple and half a cucumber into a paste to add shine and smooth texture.
- Carrot and Yogurt Mask: Blend 1 boiled carrot with ½ cup yogurt for vibrant, glossy hair.
- Beer Rinse: Use flat beer as a final rinse to enhance shine and smooth the cuticle.
- Strawberry and Olive Oil Mask: Blend 5 strawberries with 2 tbsp olive oil for a fruity shine boost.

FOR VOLUME AND THICKNESS

- Flaxseed Gel Mask: Boil 2 tbsp flaxseeds in 1 cup water, strain, and apply the gel for added body and volume.
- Egg White and Aloe Vera Mask: Beat 1 egg white with 2 tbsp aloe vera gel for thicker, fuller hair.
- Hibiscus and Coconut Oil Mask: Blend 4 hibiscus flowers with 2 tbsp coconut oil for thicker hair and fewer split ends.
- Potato Juice and Honey Mask: Combine 3 tbsp potato juice with 1 tbsp honey for plump, voluminous strands.

- Cornstarch and Coconut Oil Mask: Mix 1 tbsp cornstarch with 2 tbsp coconut oil to create a lightweight mask for lift and thickness.

How to Properly Apply a Hair Mask

To make the most of your homemade treatments, applying them correctly is essential. Here's a step-by-step guide:

Start with Clean Hair: Wash your hair with a gentle shampoo to remove dirt, oil, and product buildup. Pat your hair dry with a towel so it's damp but not dripping wet.

Section Your Hair: Divide your hair into sections to ensure the mask is evenly distributed. Clip each section away as you work.

Focus on the Right Areas:

For moisture and repair masks, concentrate on the mid-lengths and ends of your hair, as they are the most damaged.

For growth or scalp treatments, focus on massaging the mask into your scalp to stimulate blood flow and nourish the follicles.

If your hair is very dry or frizzy, apply the mask from root to tip for all-over hydration.

Massage Gently: Use your fingers to work the mask through each section, making sure every strand is coated. For scalp treatments, use circular motions to massage the product in. This not only ensures coverage but also boosts circulation, promoting healthy hair growth.

Cover Your Hair: Wrap your hair in a shower cap, plastic wrap, or a warm towel. This traps heat, helping the ingredients penetrate deeper into the hair shaft.

How Long to Keep a Hair Mask On

The time you leave a mask on depends on the ingredients and your hair's needs:

Quick Fix (10–15 Minutes): Masks with lightweight oils, yogurt, or honey work well in shorter sessions for hydration and shine.

Deep Treatments (20–30 Minutes): Masks with rich oils like coconut or castor oil, or protein-rich ingredients like eggs, need more time to work their magic.

Overnight Treatments: Some masks, especially those focused on hydration or growth, can be left on overnight for intensive care. Examples include aloe vera and coconut oil blends. Use a silk scarf or old towel to protect your pillowcase.

Tip: Always rinse thoroughly with lukewarm water after the mask. For heavy or oil-based masks, follow up with a mild shampoo to prevent residue buildup.

By following these steps, you'll maximize the benefits of your DIY treatments, giving your hair the nourishment and care it craves. The effort you put into the application process helps ensure each recipe works its wonders, leaving your hair healthier, shinier, and more vibrant.

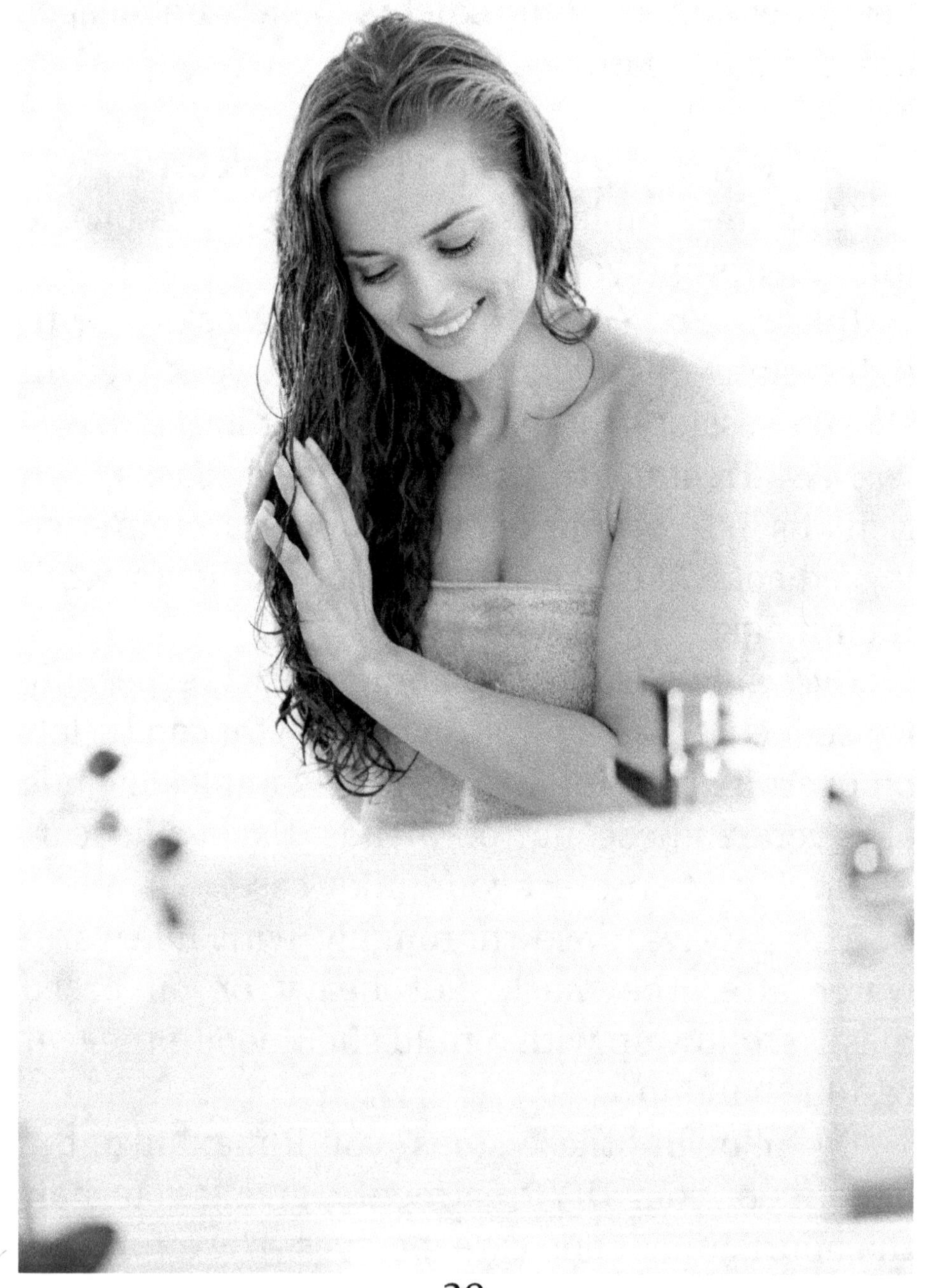

CHAPTER 5: CHOOSING THE PERFECT PRODUCTS—YOUR GUIDE TO TAILORED HAIR CARE

With so many hair care products on the market, finding the right ones can feel overwhelming. The key to selecting high-quality products lies in understanding your hair's unique characteristics—its type, structure, and needs. In this chapter, we'll guide you through choosing the best products to create a personalized hair care routine that delivers the healthy, thick, and beautiful hair you desire.

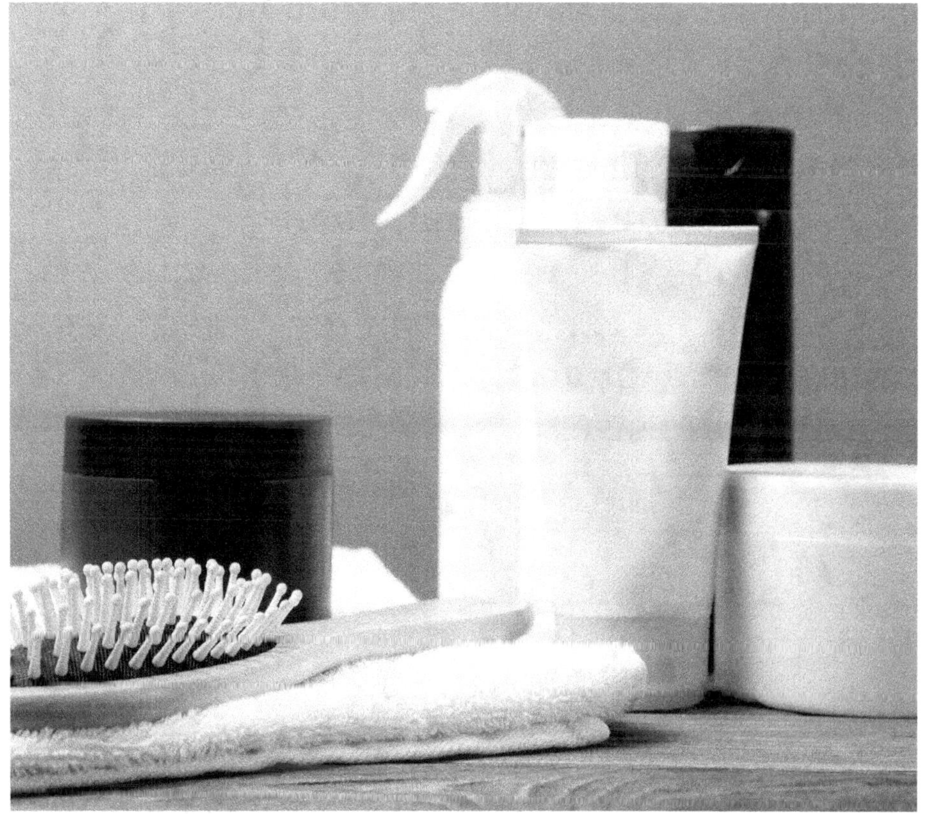

Know Your Hair Type and Structure

Before diving into products, take a moment to evaluate your hair type and structure. These factors influence what your hair needs to look and feel its best.

Hair Type:

Straight Hair: Tends to be sleek and gets oily faster because natural scalp oils travel easily down the shaft. Needs lightweight products that don't weigh it down.

Wavy Hair: Falls between straight and curly, often prone to frizz. Benefits from hydrating and frizz-control products.

Curly Hair: Naturally dry and prone to tangling because scalp oils struggle to coat the curls. Needs intense moisture and definition.

Coily Hair: The most fragile hair type, with tight curls or zigzag patterns. Needs extra nourishment, protection, and gentle care to minimize breakage.

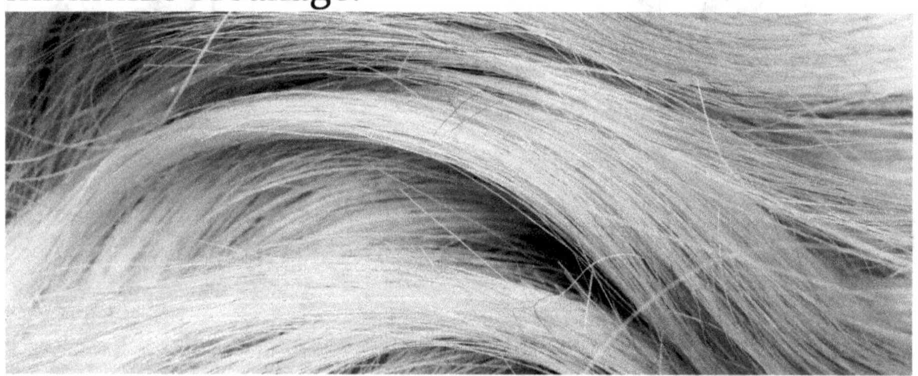

Hair Structure:

Fine Hair: Delicate strands that are easily weighed down. Needs volumizing and lightweight formulas.

Medium Hair: Versatile and can handle a wider range of products. Focus on balancing moisture and strength.

Thick Hair: Strong and often coarse, requiring rich, hydrating products to soften and tame.

What to Look for in Hair Care Products

Understanding product labels can help you identify high-quality options. Look for these key features based on your needs:

For Cleansing:

Sulfate-Free Shampoos: Sulfates strip away natural oils, so opt for gentler formulas.

Clarifying Shampoos: Use occasionally to remove product buildup, especially if you use styling products regularly.

For Moisturizing:

Hydrating Conditioners: Look for ingredients like glycerin, aloe vera, or shea butter.

Deep Conditioners: For a weekly boost of hydration and repair.

For Strengthening:

Protein-Rich Treatments: Ingredients like keratin or hydrolyzed protein fortify weak, brittle hair. Use sparingly to avoid overloading.

For Styling and Protection:

Heat Protectants: Must-have if you use heat tools; protects your hair from damage caused by high temperatures.

Leave-In Conditioners: Offer lightweight moisture and frizz control.

Serums and Oils: Add shine and tame flyaways. Look for argan oil, jojoba oil, or silicone-based serums for smoothness.

Matching Products to Your Hair Type
For Straight Hair:

Choose lightweight, oil-balancing shampoos and conditioners.

Avoid heavy creams or oils that can make hair look greasy.

Use volumizing mousses or sprays to add lift and body.

For Wavy Hair:

Use moisturizing shampoos and conditioners to reduce frizz.

Apply leave-in conditioners or curl creams to define waves without weighing them down.

A salt spray or light gel can enhance natural texture.

For Curly Hair:

Look for sulfate-free shampoos and rich, hydrating conditioners.

Opt for curl-enhancing creams or gels to

define and hold curls.

Deep condition weekly to maintain elasticity.

For Coily Hair:

Use co-washing (cleansing conditioners) to gently clean without stripping moisture.

Incorporate heavy creams, butters, and oils like shea butter or castor oil to lock in hydration.

Protective styling products help reduce breakage and preserve hair health.

How to Spot High-Quality Products
Check the Ingredient List:

Good Ingredients: Natural oils (coconut, argan, jojoba), humectants (glycerin, aloe), and proteins (keratin, silk).

Avoid: Sulfates, parabens, drying alcohols, and synthetic fragrances if you're prone to dryness or irritation.

Understand Product Labels:

Hydrating: Best for dry, frizzy, or curly hair.

Volumizing: Ideal for fine, flat hair.

Strengthening/Repairing: Designed for damaged, brittle hair.

Read Reviews: Look for products with positive feedback from people with similar hair types and concerns.

Tailoring Your Routine to Your Goals
For Growth: Look for products with biotin,

caffeine, or rosemary oil to stimulate the scalp and encourage healthy growth.

For Damage Repair: Seek out deep conditioners and masks with keratin, silk proteins, or ceramides to rebuild strength.

For Shine: Choose serums or oils with argan oil or silicone to smooth the cuticle and reflect light.

Keep It Simple

You don't need a bathroom overflowing with products to care for your hair effectively. Start with the basics—a high-quality shampoo and conditioner, a leave-in treatment, and a styling product. Build your collection gradually based on your hair's needs and the results you see.

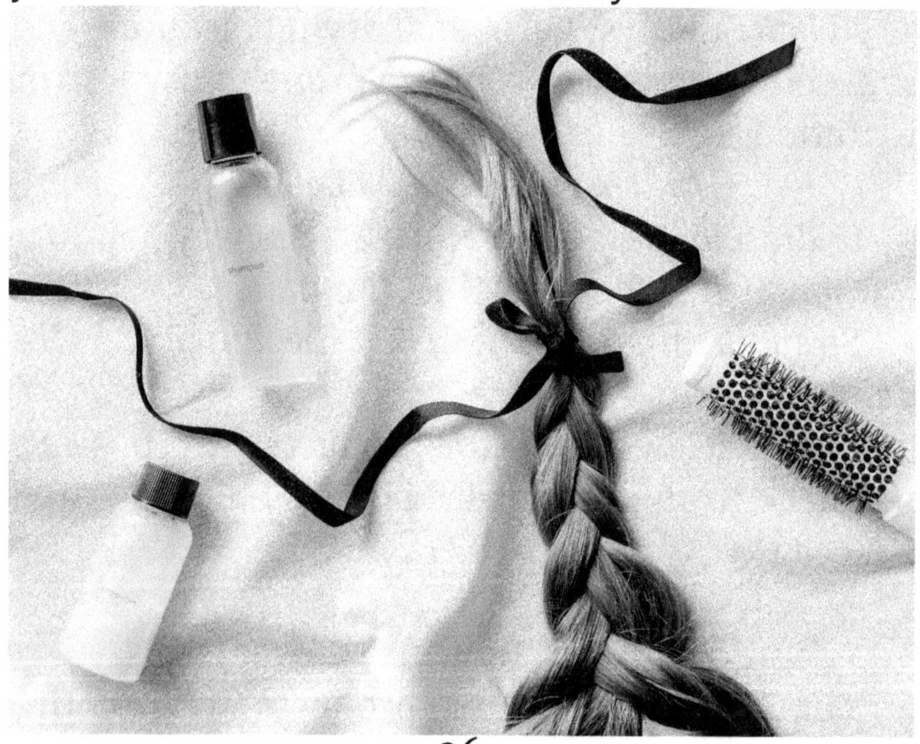

FINAL THOUGHTS: THE HAIR CARE HANDBOOK

As we reach the final pages of The Hair Care Handbook, I hope you've come to see your hair as more than just strands of protein—it's a living expression of who you are, a reflection of your care, and a source of confidence. Whether you're nurturing long, flowing locks, embracing bouncy curls, or rocking a short, sleek style, the key to achieving hair you love lies in understanding it, honoring its unique needs, and being consistent in your care.

Your Hair Journey is Unique

Throughout this book, we've explored the foundations of healthy hair care—its structure, the growth process, and the importance of choosing the right products. We've addressed common challenges like damage, frizz, and thinning, and shared recipes for natural treatments that bring luxurious care into your home.

But more than anything, we've emphasized that your hair journey is your own. It's not about chasing perfection or imitating someone else's look—it's about discovering what works for you and celebrating the beauty that's already yours.

Consistency is the Secret Ingredient

The biggest transformations happen over time. Regular trims, nourishing masks, scalp massages, and smart product choices may seem small, but together, they create a foundation of strength and resilience. Stick to the routines and habits you've discovered here, and trust the process—even when results feel slow. Hair care is a long game, and the rewards are worth the wait.

A Final Word on Self-Care

Taking care of your hair is about more than just looking good—it's about feeling good, too. The time you spend nurturing your hair is an act of self-love, a moment to pause and care for yourself. Let it be a reminder that you deserve attention, kindness, and time to feel your best.

Your Best Hair Days Are Ahead

This is not the end of your hair care journey—it's just the beginning. Keep experimenting, learning, and refining your routine as your hair's needs evolve. Embrace every phase of your journey with confidence, patience, and joy.

Here's to gorgeous, strong, and luscious locks—and the beautiful, radiant woman who wears them with pride.

Thank you for letting this book be part of your story. Your hair is your crown—wear it boldly, beautifully, and unapologetically.

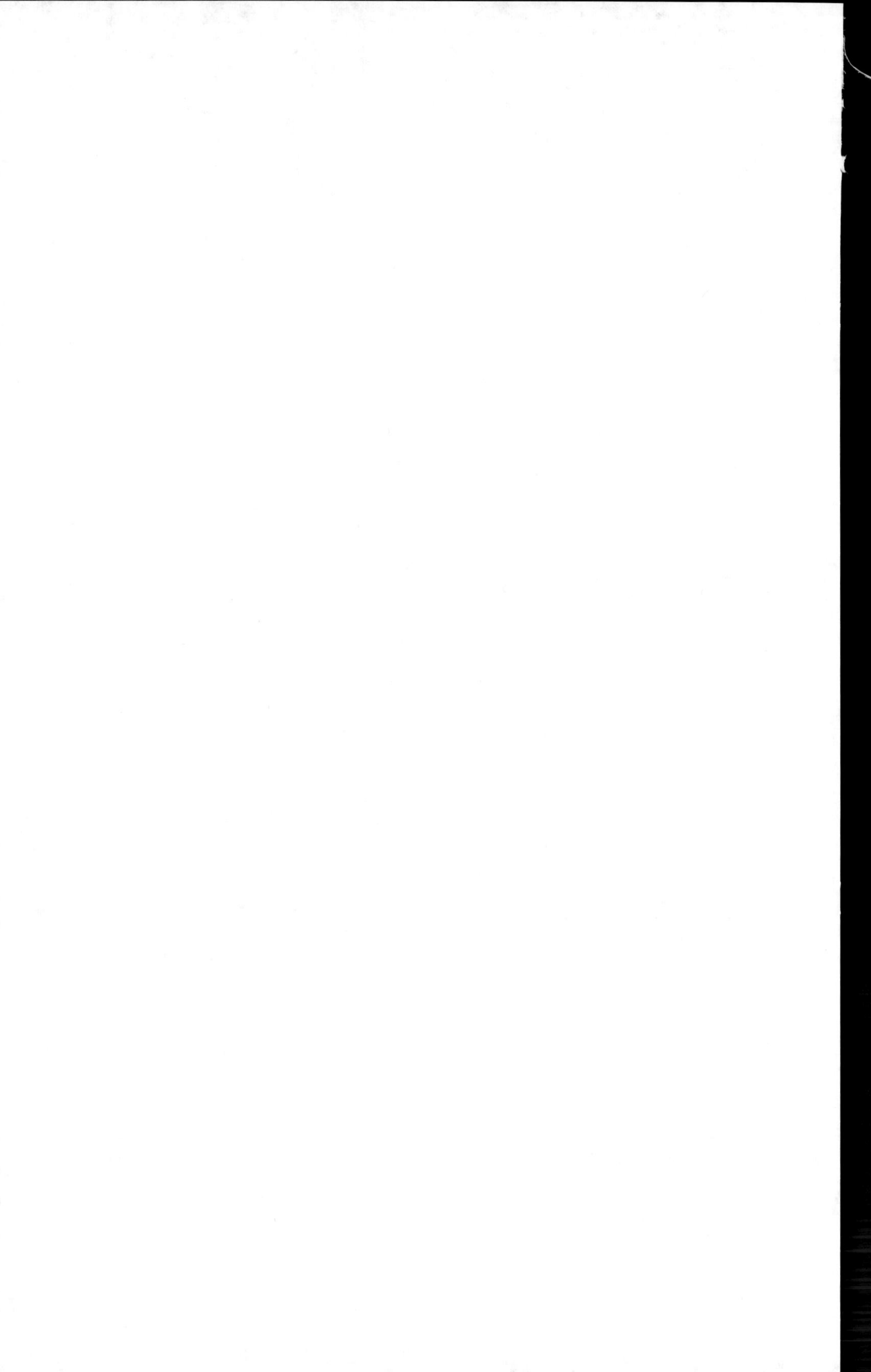